TRANSGENDER JOURNEY:

Understanding Identity and Equality

Sabat Beatto

Dedication

This book is dedicated to the vibrant and resilient LGBTQ+ community worldwide. It is a testament to your courage, strength, and unwavering pursuit of authenticity. You inspire us all with your unwavering commitment to embracing your true selves and advocating for equality.

To those who have embarked on their own transgender journey, this dedication is a tribute to your bravery in navigating the complexities of identity. May this book serve as a beacon of understanding, support, and empowerment as you explore and embrace your authentic selves.

To the countless allies who stand alongside the LGBTQ+ community, your unwavering support and acceptance have made a profound impact. This dedication acknowledges your commitment to inclusivity and your tireless efforts to promote equality and celebrate diversity.

May the pages of this book serve as a testament to our shared humanity, a reminder that every individual deserves respect, understanding, and equal rights. Together, let us continue to create a world that embraces and celebrates the beauty of diverse identities.

Table of Contents

Introduction 1

Chapter 2: Understanding Transgenderism: Definitions
and Concepts..3

Chapter 3: Historical Perspective: Transgender Rights Movements......5

Chapter 4: Basic Human Freedom and Individual Choice 7

Chapter 5: Pre-Sexual Development: The Formation of
Gender Identity..9

Chapter 6: Sexual Orientation: Exploring Diverse Attractions 11

Chapter 7: Biological Sex and Gender: Differentiating Between
the Two 13

Chapter 8: The Dark Side of Transgender Individuals:
Stigmatization and Discrimination... 15

Chapter 9: Mental Health and Transgender Individuals:
Challenges and Resilience... 19

Chapter 10: Transgender Medicine: Hormonal and Surgical
Interventions 23

Chapter 11: Gender Identity Disorder: Diagnostic Criteria
and Controversies.. 27

Chapter 12: Ethical Considerations in Transgender Healthcare 29

Chapter 13: Rushing to Operate: The Risks and Benefits of
Gender-Affirming Surgeries 33

Chapter 14: Supporting Transgender Youth: Education and
Mental Health 37

Chapter 15: The Role of Family and Social Support in Transgender Lives 41

Chapter 16: Transgender Rights and Legal Protections 45

Chapter 17: Intersectionality: Exploring the Experiences of Transgender People of Color 49

Chapter 18: Media Representation and Its Impact on Transgender Individuals 53

Chapter 19: Religion and Transgender Issues: Perspectives and Conflicts 57

Chapter 20: Debunking Myths: Addressing Misconceptions about Transgender People 61

Chapter 21: Lack of Real Science: Examining Controversial Research and Debates 65

Chapter 22: Transgender in the Workplace: Challenges and Progress 69

Chapter 23: Transgender and Sports: Fairness and Inclusion 71

Chapter 24: Transgender Activism: Milestones and Current Movements 75

Chapter 25: Gender-Affirming Care for Non-Binary and Gender-Fluid Individuals 79

Chapter 26: Transgender Rights on a Global Scale 83

Chapter 27: Mental Health Support for Transgender Individuals 87

Chapter 28: The Role of Allies in the Transgender Rights Movement 91

Chapter 29: Future Directions: Advancements and Challenges 95

Conclusion: Towards a More Inclusive and Understanding Society 99

This outline covers various topics related to the transgender agenda, highlighting various perspectives, controversies, challenges, and progress in understanding and supporting transgender individuals.

Introduction

In recent years, discussions surrounding gender identity, sexual orientation, and the transgender agenda have become increasingly prevalent. As understanding these complex issues evolves, engaging in open and informed conversations exploring the multifaceted aspects of these topics is important. This book delves into the intricacies of the transgender agenda, highlighting the fundamental principles of basic human freedom and individual choice that underpin these discussions.

At the core of the transgender agenda is recognizing the diversity of human experiences and the right of individuals to express their gender identity authentically. Throughout history, transgender individuals have faced significant challenges in accessing equal rights and facing societal acceptance. Understanding their struggles, triumphs, and the social movements that have fought for their rights is essential in cultivating empathy and fostering an inclusive society.

As we embark on this exploration, we will delve into various dimensions of transgender issues, starting with examining the basic concepts and definitions that form the foundation of our understanding. We will navigate through the complexities of pre-sexual development, exploring how gender identity forms and the different factors that shape it. Additionally, we will explore sexual orientation, recognizing the diverse range of attractions that individuals experience.

While acknowledging the importance of individual choice and freedom, it is crucial to address the challenges faced by transgender individuals. Stigmatization, Discrimination, and the dark side of these issues demand our attention and efforts toward creating a more equitable society. Mental health considerations, the role of family and social support, and legal protections for transgender individuals will also be examined to provide a comprehensive understanding of their challenges.

Furthermore, this book sheds light on the medical aspects of transgenderism, including hormonal and surgical interventions, ethical considerations in transgender healthcare, and the controversies surrounding gender identity disorder diagnosis. We will critically evaluate the rush to undergo gender-affirming surgeries, emphasizing the importance of informed decision-making and comprehensive care.

However, it is equally important to acknowledge some concerns regarding the transgender agenda. This book will explore the lack of real science behind certain claims and controversies, ensuring a balanced perspective that examines multiple viewpoints. Doing so can foster an environment that encourages open dialogue and evidence-based discussions.

Ultimately, this book aims to provide a comprehensive and nuanced exploration of the transgender agenda, human freedom, individual choices, and the underlying scientific and social complexities. By delving into these topics, we hope to contribute to a more inclusive and understanding society that embraces the rights and experiences of transgender individuals. Let us embark on this journey together, seeking knowledge, empathy, and positive change.

Chapter 2: Understanding Transgenderism: Definitions and Concepts

Transgenderism is a complex and multifaceted aspect of human identity that challenges traditional understandings of gender. In this chapter, we will explore the definitions and concepts that form the foundation of our understanding of transgenderism.

1. Defining Transgender:

- Transgender refers to individuals whose gender identity does not align with the sex assigned to them at birth. They may identify as a gender different from the one typically associated with their biological sex.
- It is important to distinguish between gender identity and sexual orientation. Gender identity pertains to one's internal sense of being male, female, or another gender, while sexual orientation relates to one's attraction to others.

2. Gender Dysphoria:

- Gender dysphoria is psychological distress experienced by some transgender individuals due to the incongruence between their assigned sex and gender identity.
- The diagnostic term "gender identity disorder" was used in the past. Still, it has been replaced by "gender dysphoria" in the Diagnostic and Statistical Manual of Mental Disorders (DSM-5), reflecting a shift towards depathologizing transgender identities.

3. Gender Expression:

- Gender expression refers to the outward manifestation of one's gender identity through behavior, clothing, hairstyle, and other external cues.
- Transgender individuals may express their gender identity differently from societal expectations of their assigned sex.

4. Non-Binary and Gender-Fluid Identities:

- Non-binary and gender-fluid individuals do not exclusively identify as male or female. They may experience a fluidity of gender identity or identify outside the traditional binary framework.
- Recognizing and respecting non-binary and gender-fluid identities is essential for creating inclusive spaces for all individuals.

5. Transitioning:

- Transitioning refers to how transgender individuals align their gender expression, physical appearance, and social roles with their gender identity.
- Transitioning may involve social changes, such as coming out and changing one's name and pronouns, and medical interventions, such as hormone therapy or gender-affirming surgeries.

6. Intersectionality:

- Intersectionality recognizes that transgender individuals can face additional discrimination and marginalization based on race, ethnicity, class, disability, or immigration status.
- Understanding the interconnectedness of various social identities is crucial for addressing the diverse experiences and needs of transgender individuals.

As we delve into these definitions and concepts, we must approach transgenderism with empathy, respect, and a willingness to learn. Recognizing the complexity of gender identity and the experiences of transgender individuals is essential for fostering inclusivity and promoting understanding.

Chapter 3: Historical Perspective: Transgender Rights Movements

The struggle for transgender rights has a rich and complex history that spans several decades. This chapter provides an overview of the key milestones and movements that have shaped the advancement of transgender rights.

1. Stonewall Riots and the Birth of the Modern LGBTQ+ Movement:

- The Stonewall Riots in June 1969 in New York City were pivotal in the fight for LGBTQ+ rights.
- While primarily known for its impact on gay rights, the riots also played a significant role in mobilizing transgender individuals, who were at the forefront of the resistance against police harassment and discrimination.

2. Transgender Activism in the 20th Century:

- In the 20th century, transgender activists began organizing and advocating for their rights and visibility.
- Pioneers such as Marsha P. Johnson and Sylvia Rivera played crucial roles in raising awareness about transgender issues and fighting for equality.

3. Legal Recognition and Protection:

- In the late 20th and early 21st centuries, legal battles for transgender rights gained traction.

- Landmark legal cases, such as M.T. v. J.T. (2000) and the Supreme Court's ruling in Obergefell v. Hodges (2015), helped to advance legal recognition of transgender individuals and their right to gender-affirming documentation and marriage equality.

4. Evolving Terminology and Language:

- The language and terminology surrounding transgender identities and rights have evolved.

- From the medical pathologization of transgender identities to adopting more affirming terms like "gender identity" and "gender expression," language has significantly shaped public perception and policy changes.

5. Global Transgender Rights Movements:

- Transgender rights movements are not limited to one country or region.

- Activists and organizations worldwide have been working on challenging discriminatory laws, advocating for legal recognition, and promoting social acceptance of transgender individuals.

6. Transgender Visibility in Media and Culture:

- Increased visibility of transgender individuals in media, including TV shows, films, and documentaries, has helped raise awareness and challenge stereotypes.

- Cultural moments, such as actress Laverne Cox's portrayal of a transgender character in "Orange Is the New Black," have contributed to shifting societal perceptions.

Understanding the historical context of transgender rights movements allows us to appreciate the progress made, as well as the ongoing challenges faced by transgender individuals. It highlights the resilience, strength, and determination of activists who have paved the way for greater acceptance and recognition of transgender rights.

Chapter 4: Basic Human Freedom and Individual Choice

Fundamental to the discussion of transgenderism and related issues is the recognition of basic human freedom and the importance of individual choice. This chapter explores the principles and implications of these concepts.

1. Autonomy and Self-Determination:

- Basic human freedom encompasses the principles of autonomy and self-determination, affirming an individual's right to choose their own life, identity, and body.

- Respecting autonomy means acknowledging that individuals can define and express their gender identity and make decisions about their gender-affirming care.

2. Inclusive Society and Personal Freedom:

- An inclusive society values personal freedom and recognizes that diverse identities and expressions should be embraced and celebrated.

- Allowing individuals to explore and express their gender identity without fear of discrimination or judgment promotes personal freedom and a more inclusive society.

3. Challenging Social Norms and Expectations:

- Embracing individual choice entails challenging societal norms and expectations regarding gender roles and expressions.

- By questioning and breaking free from rigid gender stereotypes, individuals can exercise their freedom to authentically express their gender identity.

4. Intersectionality and Multiple Identities:

- Recognizing and respecting individual choice means understanding that individuals have intersecting identities and experiences.

Chapter 5: Pre-Sexual Development: The Formation of Gender Identity

The development of gender identity begins long before sexual maturity and involves a complex interplay of biological, psychological, and social factors. This chapter explores the pre-sexual development process and sheds light on the formation of gender identity.

1. Nature and Nurture:

- Both biological and environmental factors influence the formation of gender identity. Biological factors include genetic and hormonal influences, while environmental factors encompass socialization, cultural norms, and familial upbringing.

2. Early Childhood and Gender Socialization:

- Gender socialization starts early in childhood, as children are exposed to societal expectations and stereotypes associated with gender.
- Family, peers, media, and educational institutions significantly shape a child's understanding of gender roles, behaviors, and expressions.

3. Gender Typing and Cognition:

- Gender typing refers to how children learn and understand gender roles and expectations.
- Cognitive development, such as forming gender schemas, contributes to how children perceive themselves and others regarding gender.

4. Gender Identity Formation:

- Around two or three, children develop a sense of gender identity.
- Gender identity is the deeply felt sense of being male, female, or another gender. It may align with the sex assigned at birth (cisgender) or differ from it (transgender).

5. Gender Identity Stability and Constancy:

- As children age, their gender identity becomes more stable and consistent.
- By age six or seven, most children clearly and consistently understand their gender identity, which often aligns with their assigned sex.

6. Exploration and Nonconforming Identities:

- Some children may question or explore gender identities that differ from societal expectations.
- Gender-nonconforming children may exhibit behaviors, preferences, or expressions that do not align with typical gender stereotypes.

7. Supportive Environments:

- Creating supportive and affirming environments for children's gender exploration is crucial.
- Families, schools, and communities can play a pivotal role in fostering an inclusive atmosphere that respects and affirms children's gender identities.

Understanding the pre-sexual development process helps us appreciate the complexity and individuality of gender identity formation. Recognizing the influence of various factors and supporting children in their gender exploration can contribute to their well-being and self-acceptance.

Chapter 6: Sexual Orientation: Exploring Diverse Attractions

Sexual orientation refers to an individual's enduring pattern of emotional, romantic, and/or sexual attraction to others. This chapter delves into the concept of sexual orientation, highlighting the diverse range of attractions people experience.

1. Understanding Sexual Orientation:

- Sexual orientation is a fundamental aspect of human identity and encompasses a spectrum of attractions.
- The three main categories of sexual orientation are heterosexual (attraction to people of the opposite gender), homosexual (attraction to people of the same gender), and bisexual (attraction to people of both the same and opposite genders).

2. Fluidity and Spectrum:

- Sexual orientation exists on a spectrum, with individuals experiencing different degrees of attraction and flexibility over time.
- Some individuals may identify as exclusively heterosexual, homosexual, or bisexual, while others may identify as queer, pansexual, or asexual, among other identities.

3. Coming Out and Self-Acceptance:

- Coming out refers to revealing one's sexual orientation to others, often accompanied by self-acceptance and self-disclosure.

- Coming out can be a transformative and empowering experience, enabling individuals to live authentically and seek supportive communities.

Chapter 7: Biological Sex and Gender: Differentiating Between the Two

Biological sex and gender are distinct but interconnected concepts. This chapter explores the differences between biological sex and gender, highlighting the complexities of these terms.

1. Biological Sex:

- Biological sex refers to the physical and physiological attributes that typically distinguish males from females.

- Various factors, including reproductive anatomy, chromosomes, hormones, and secondary sexual characteristics, determine it.

2. Chromosomes and Gonads:

- Chromosomes play a significant role in determining biological sex. Typically, males have one X and Y chromosome (XY), while females have two X chromosomes (XX).

- Gonads, such as testes or ovaries, develop in response to the chromosomal makeup and influence the production of sex hormones.

3. Secondary Sexual Characteristics:

- Secondary sexual characteristics, such as breast development, facial hair, or voice pitch, emerge during puberty and are influenced by sex hormones.

- These characteristics are often associated with and used to differentiate between males and females in a given society.

4. Gender:

- Gender refers to the socially and culturally constructed roles, behaviors, and expectations of being male or female.
- It is a complex and multifaceted concept encompassing personal identity, expression, and societal norms.

5. Gender Identity:

- Gender identity refers to an individual's deeply felt sense of being male, female, or another gender.
- It may or may not align with the sex assigned at birth. Some individuals identify as cisgender, where their gender identity aligns with their assigned sex, while others identify as transgender.

6. Gender Expression:

- Gender expression refers to how individuals present their gender to others through clothing, hairstyles, behaviors, and other external cues.
- Gender expression can vary greatly and may not necessarily align with societal expectations based on biological sex.

7. Gender Roles and Expectations:

- Gender roles are the social expectations and norms of being male or female in a particular culture or society.
- These roles can influence behavior, occupations, relationships, and societal expectations placed on individuals.

Understanding the distinction between biological sex and gender is crucial for recognizing and respecting individuals' diverse experiences and identities. It helps challenge societal stereotypes and allows for a more inclusive and nuanced understanding of human diversity.

Chapter 8: The Dark Side of Transgender Individuals: Stigmatization and Discrimination

Transgender individuals often face significant challenges and discrimination in various aspects of their lives. This chapter sheds light on the dark side of transgender experiences, including stigmatization and discrimination.

1. Stigmatization:

- Stigmatization refers to society's negative attitudes, stereotypes, and prejudices toward transgender individuals.
- Transphobia, which encompasses fear, prejudice, and hostility towards transgender people, contributes to their stigmatization.

2. Discrimination and Marginalization:

- Transgender individuals often face discrimination and marginalization in different spheres of life, including education, employment, housing, healthcare, and legal systems.
- They may be denied equal opportunities, face harassment, and experience unequal treatment due to gender identity.

3. Violence and Hate Crimes:

- Transgender individuals are at a heightened risk of experiencing violence and hate crimes.

- Transphobic violence, including physical assault, sexual violence, and murder, is a severe consequence of the prejudice and discrimination faced by transgender individuals.

4. Mental Health Challenges:

- Stigmatization and discrimination can have significant mental health impacts on transgender individuals.
- Higher rates of depression, anxiety, self-harm, and suicide attempts are observed among transgender individuals, highlighting the toll of societal rejection and prejudice.

5. Healthcare Disparities:

- Transgender individuals often face barriers to accessing competent and inclusive healthcare.
- Discrimination from healthcare providers, lack of understanding, and limited access to gender-affirming care can harm their well-being.

6. Legal Challenges:

- Legal recognition and protection for transgender individuals vary across jurisdictions.
- Many transgender individuals face challenges in obtaining legal recognition of their gender identity, changing identification documents, and accessing legal protections against discrimination.

7. Intersectionality and Multiple Forms of Discrimination:

- Transgender individuals who belong to marginalized communities based on race, ethnicity, socioeconomic status, or disability often face intersecting forms of discrimination.
- Intersectionality further exacerbates the challenges they experience and requires a comprehensive understanding of the multiple layers of discrimination they face.

Understanding the dark side of transgender experiences is crucial for promoting empathy, raising awareness, and advocating for change. Combatting stigmatization and discrimination requires collective efforts to create inclusive societies that recognize and respect the rights and dignity of all individuals, regardless of their gender identity.

CHAPTER 8

Chapter 9: Mental Health and Transgender Individuals: Challenges and Resilience

Transgender individuals often face unique mental health challenges due to the stigma, discrimination, and societal pressures they encounter. However, many also demonstrate remarkable resilience in navigating these challenges. This chapter explores the mental health experiences of transgender individuals, highlighting both the difficulties and their capacity for resilience.

1. Mental Health Disparities:

- Transgender individuals are at a higher risk for mental health issues than the general population.
- Factors such as stigma, discrimination, minority stress, social isolation, and lack of access to affirmative healthcare contribute to these disparities.

2. Gender Dysphoria:

- Gender dysphoria is clinically significant distress arising from the incongruence between a person's gender identity and their assigned sex at birth.
- Gender-affirming interventions, such as hormone therapy and gender-confirming surgeries, can alleviate gender dysphoria and improve mental well-being.

3. Depression and Anxiety:

- Transgender individuals experience higher rates of depression and anxiety disorders than the general population.

- These conditions may result from minority stress, internalized transphobia, social rejection, and the challenges associated with gender transition.

4. Suicidal Ideation and Self-Harm:

- Transgender individuals face an elevated risk of suicidal ideation and self-harm.

- The combination of societal stigma, discrimination, and lack of support can contribute to feelings of hopelessness and desperation.

5. Resilience and Coping Strategies:

- Despite the challenges, many transgender individuals exhibit remarkable resilience and demonstrate effective coping strategies.

- Building social support networks, seeking gender-affirming healthcare, finding community, and embracing self-acceptance can contribute to resilience and improved mental well-being.

6. Mental Health Care and Support:

- Accessible and affirming mental health care is essential for transgender individuals.

- Mental health professionals who are knowledgeable about transgender issues, culturally competent, and sensitive to the unique needs of this population can provide invaluable support.

7. Empowering Narratives and Visibility:

- Increasing transgender visibility and positive representation in media and society can play a crucial role in promoting mental health and resilience.

- Sharing diverse narratives and stories of transgender individuals can help combat stigma, promote understanding, and inspire others.

Recognizing the mental health challenges faced by transgender individuals is vital for fostering supportive environments and improving access to appropriate care. By promoting resilience, empowerment, and understanding, we can contribute to better mental well-being and support the flourishing of transgender individuals.

Chapter 10: Transgender Medicine: Hormonal and Surgical Interventions

Transgender medicine encompasses a range of medical interventions to align an individual's physical body with their gender identity. This chapter explores the two primary interventions: hormonal therapy and surgical procedures.

1. Hormonal Therapy:

- Hormonal therapy, also known as hormone replacement therapy (HRT), involves the administration of hormones to induce changes that align with an individual's gender identity.

- For transgender women (assigned male at birth), feminizing hormones such as estrogen and anti-androgens are prescribed to promote breast development, decrease body hair growth, and induce other secondary sexual characteristics.

- For transgender men (assigned female at birth), masculinizing hormones such as testosterone are administered to promote voice deepening, facial and body hair growth, and other masculine secondary sexual characteristics.

2. Mental Health Evaluation and Hormonal Therapy:

- Before starting hormonal therapy, individuals typically undergo a comprehensive mental health evaluation.

- The evaluation helps ensure that individuals understand hormonal therapy's effects and potential risks and are mentally prepared for the physical changes they will experience.

3. Surgical Interventions:

- Surgical interventions, often referred to as gender-affirming surgeries or sex reassignment surgeries, are options for some transgender individuals who desire permanent physical changes.
- For transgender women, surgical procedures may include breast augmentation, facial feminization surgery, or genital reconstruction surgery (vaginoplasty).
- For transgender men, surgical procedures may include chest masculinization (top surgery), genital reconstruction surgery (phalloplasty or metoidioplasty), or hysterectomy and oophorectomy (removal of the uterus and ovaries).

4. Eligibility and Access:

- Eligibility for surgical interventions varies depending on age, mental health evaluation, and specific healthcare guidelines or criteria.
- Geographical location, financial resources, healthcare policies, and availability of trained surgeons may influence access to gender-affirming surgeries.

5. Comprehensive Care and Multidisciplinary Approach:

- Transgender medicine emphasizes a comprehensive and multidisciplinary approach to care.
- This includes collaboration between medical professionals, mental health providers, and supportive care teams to ensure individuals receive appropriate medical interventions, psychosocial support, and follow-up care.

6. Potential Benefits and Risks:

- Hormonal and surgical interventions can significantly positively affect the well-being and quality of life of many transgender individuals.

- However, like any medical intervention, potential risks and side effects should be discussed thoroughly with healthcare professionals.

Transgender medicine, including hormonal and surgical interventions, aims to assist transgender individuals in aligning their physical bodies with their gender identity. Access to comprehensive and affirming care is crucial in supporting the overall well-being and happiness of transgender individuals.

Chapter 11: Gender Identity Disorder: Diagnostic Criteria and Controversies

Gender identity disorder, now known as gender dysphoria, was a diagnostic category used in the past to describe individuals whose gender identity did not align with their assigned sex at birth. This chapter explores the diagnostic criteria associated with gender identity disorder and examines the controversies surrounding its classification.

1. Diagnostic Criteria:

- The diagnostic criteria for gender identity disorder, as outlined in previous versions of the Diagnostic and Statistical Manual of Mental Disorders (DSM), included a persistent and strong desire to be the other gender and significant distress caused by the incongruence between gender identity and assigned sex.

- Individuals had to exhibit these feelings and experiences for at least six months to meet the diagnostic criteria.

2. Gender Dysphoria:

- In more recent editions of the DSM, the term "gender identity disorder" has been replaced by "gender dysphoria."

- Gender dysphoria reflects a shift in understanding, recognizing that distress arises from the incongruence between gender identity and assigned sex rather than the gender identity itself.

3. Controversies and Criticisms:

- The inclusion of gender dysphoria in the DSM and its classification as a mental disorder has been the subject of ongoing debate and criticism.
- Some argue that pathologizing gender diversity contributes to stigma and hinders access to necessary healthcare and legal protections for transgender individuals.

4. Gender Diversity as a Natural Variation:

- Many advocates and healthcare professionals argue that gender diversity is a natural variation of human experience rather than a disorder.
- They assert that gender dysphoria should be approached from a framework of understanding and acceptance rather than pathology.

5. Evolving Perspectives:

- The understanding of gender identity and its relationship with mental health is evolving.
- There is a growing recognition of the importance of providing gender-affirming care and support to transgender individuals rather than focusing on diagnostic labels.

6. Access to Gender-Affirming Care:

- Despite the controversies surrounding the diagnosis, including gender dysphoria in the DSM, it has facilitated access to gender-affirming healthcare for many transgender individuals.
- It has provided a framework for healthcare professionals to provide necessary interventions, such as hormone therapy and gender-confirming surgeries.

As perspectives on gender identity and mental health continue to evolve, it is important to critically examine the diagnostic criteria associated with gender dysphoria and ensure that healthcare practices and policies promote the well-being and self-determination of transgender individuals.

Chapter 12: Ethical Considerations in Transgender Healthcare

Transgender healthcare raises important ethical considerations that healthcare professionals and society must address. This chapter explores key ethical considerations in providing healthcare to transgender individuals.

1. Autonomy and Informed Consent:

- Respecting the autonomy of transgender individuals is essential. Healthcare providers should involve patients in decision-making regarding their care and ensure informed consent for medical interventions.

- Informed consent should include a thorough discussion of the potential risks, benefits, and alternatives, allowing individuals to make well-informed decisions about their gender-affirming care.

2. Non-Discrimination and Equal Treatment:

- Transgender individuals can receive healthcare without discrimination, prejudice, or bias.

- Healthcare providers should strive to provide equitable and inclusive care, regardless of a person's gender identity or expression.

3. Gender-Affirming Care:

- The principle of providing gender-affirming care emphasizes meeting the unique healthcare needs of transgender individuals and supporting their gender identity.

- This includes access to hormone therapy, gender-confirming surgeries, mental health support, and other necessary interventions.

4. Mental Health Support:

- Mental health support is crucial for transgender individuals, particularly those experiencing gender dysphoria or navigating gender transition.
- Healthcare providers should offer accessible and affirming mental health services, including counseling, therapy, and support groups.

5. Confidentiality and Privacy:

- Respecting the confidentiality and privacy of transgender individuals is paramount.
- Healthcare providers should safeguard sensitive medical information and create a safe environment for open and honest communication.

6. Cultural Competence and Education:

- Healthcare professionals should strive to enhance their cultural competence and understanding of transgender issues.
- Continuing education and training can help providers develop the knowledge and skills to provide compassionate and effective care to transgender individuals.

7. Intersectionality and Inclusivity:

- Recognizing the intersectionality of transgender identities and experiences is crucial.
- Healthcare should address the unique needs and challenges faced by transgender individuals who belong to marginalized communities based on race, ethnicity, socioeconomic status, or disability.

8. Research and Evidence-Based Practices:

- Research on transgender healthcare is essential for advancing evidence-based practices.

- Ethical research should prioritize the well-being of transgender individuals, avoid exploitation, and strive for inclusivity.

Addressing these ethical considerations is vital for promoting equitable, compassionate, and effective healthcare for transgender individuals. By upholding principles of autonomy, non-discrimination, gender affirmation, and cultural competence, healthcare providers can contribute to the well-being and empowerment of transgender individuals.

CHAPTER 12

Chapter 13: Rushing to Operate: The Risks and Benefits of Gender-Affirming Surgeries

Gender-affirming surgeries are an important component of transgender healthcare, but it is crucial to carefully consider the risks and benefits associated with these procedures. This chapter explores the potential consequences of rushing into gender-affirming surgeries without proper evaluation and preparation.

1. Comprehensive Assessment and Mental Health Evaluation:

- Before undergoing gender-affirming surgeries, individuals should undergo a comprehensive mental health evaluation.

- Thorough evaluation helps ensure that individuals are mentally prepared, have a realistic understanding of the risks and benefits, and have explored alternative options.

2. Physical Health and Surgical Risks:

- Like any surgical procedure, gender-affirming surgeries carry inherent risks such as complications, scarring, infection, and anesthesia-related risks.

- Pre-existing medical conditions or certain medications may increase surgical risks and must be considered before proceeding.

3. Psychological Preparation and Adjustment:

- Gender-affirming surgeries can have profound psychological impacts on individuals.

- Rushing into surgery without sufficient time for adjustment and psychological preparation may lead to unrealistic expectations, dissatisfaction, or regret.

4. Postoperative Recovery and Support:

- Gender-affirming surgeries often require a significant recovery, during which individuals may experience pain, discomfort, and physical limitations.
- Adequate postoperative support, including access to pain management, wound care, and mental health support, is crucial for a successful recovery.

5. Impact on Fertility and Reproductive Options:

- Some gender-affirming surgeries may impact fertility and reproductive options.
- Individuals should be counseled about these potential consequences and provided with information about fertility preservation options before surgery, especially if they desire biological children.

6. Emotional and Social Adjustments:

- Gender-affirming surgeries can lead to emotional and social adjustments, both positive and challenging.
- Individuals may experience relationships, social interactions, and self-perception changes, which require ongoing support and adjustment.

7. Patient-Centered Decision-Making:

- Healthcare providers must engage in patient-centered decision-making, prioritizing the needs and preferences of individuals seeking gender-affirming surgeries.
- Open and honest communication, informed consent, and shared decision-making processes can help individuals make well-informed choices about their healthcare.

8. Long-Term Satisfaction and Quality of Life:

- While gender-affirming surgeries can positively impact individuals' quality of life, it is crucial to consider the long-term satisfaction and potential challenges that may arise.

- Continued follow-up care, mental health support, and resource access are important for optimizing long-term outcomes.

Balancing the risks and benefits of gender-affirming surgeries requires a careful and individualized approach. Healthcare providers should collaborate with individuals seeking surgery, ensuring they are well-informed, supported, and prepared for the physical, emotional, and social changes accompanying these procedures.

Chapter 14: Supporting Transgender Youth: Education and Mental Health

Transgender youth face unique challenges and require supportive environments to thrive. This chapter explores the importance of education and mental health support in promoting the well-being and success of transgender youth.

1. Creating Inclusive School Environments:

- Schools play a crucial role in supporting transgender youth. Creating inclusive environments fosters a sense of belonging, safety, and acceptance.

- Implementing policies that address gender identity, using preferred names and pronouns, and providing gender-neutral facilities are key steps toward inclusivity.

2. Gender-Affirming Education:

- Incorporating gender-affirming education into school curricula promotes understanding, empathy, and acceptance of transgender youth.

- Educating students, teachers, and administrators about transgender issues, identities, and experiences help combat stigma and discrimination.

3. Anti-Bullying and Supportive Policies:

- Schools should have comprehensive anti-bullying policies that explicitly address bullying based on gender identity.

- Providing resources and support networks, such as LGBTQ+ student organizations or support groups, helps create a sense of community and belonging.

4. Mental Health Support Services:

- Accessible and affirming mental health services are crucial for transgender youth.
- School counselors, psychologists, or social workers should be trained to address the specific needs of transgender youth and provide appropriate support.

5. Providing Gender-Affirming Healthcare:

- Schools can support transgender youth by advocating for gender-affirming healthcare services, such as access to puberty blockers and hormone therapy.
- Collaborating with healthcare professionals and parents/guardians helps ensure comprehensive care for transgender youth.

6. Supportive Family and Community Engagement:

- Supporting transgender youth requires engagement with families and communities.
- Providing resources, educational materials, and support groups for parents/guardians helps create a supportive network and fosters understanding and acceptance.

7. Respecting Privacy and Confidentiality:

- Respecting the privacy and confidentiality of transgender youth is essential.
- School staff should be trained to handle sensitive information with discretion and ensure the safety and well-being of transgender students.

8. Preventing and Addressing Discrimination:

- Schools must actively work to prevent and address discrimination against transgender youth.
- Enforcing non-discrimination policies, promoting a culture of acceptance, and addressing incidents of discrimination are vital steps in creating a safe and inclusive environment.

By prioritizing education, promoting mental health support, and fostering inclusive and supportive environments, schools can play a critical role in the well-being and success of transgender youth. Collaborative efforts involving educators, healthcare professionals, families, and communities are key to creating environments where transgender youth can thrive and reach their full potential.

Chapter 15: The Role of Family and Social Support in Transgender Lives

Family and social support are crucial for the well-being and resilience of transgender individuals. This chapter explores the importance of supportive families and inclusive social networks in the lives of transgender individuals.

1. Family Acceptance:

- Acceptance and support from family members significantly impact the mental health and overall well-being of transgender individuals.

- Families can play a crucial role in affirming and validating their transgender loved one's gender identity, fostering a sense of belonging, and reducing the risk of negative mental health outcomes.

2. Education and Communication:

- Families benefit from education and resources that enhance their understanding of transgender issues and experiences.

- Open and honest communication within the family creates a safe space for transgender individuals to express their needs and feelings.

3. Building Resilient Support Networks:

- Supportive social networks beyond the family are essential for transgender individuals.

- Friends, peers, and chosen family can provide understanding, acceptance, and a sense of community, helping transgender individuals navigate challenges and celebrate their identities.

4. Advocacy and Allyship:

- Families and social networks can actively advocate for transgender rights and inclusivity.
- By becoming allies, they create a more accepting society and challenge stigma and discrimination.

5. Mental Health Support:

- Providing access to mental health support is crucial for transgender individuals and their families.
- Support groups, counseling, and therapy can help address the unique challenges and promote emotional well-being.

6. Celebrating Gender Diversity:

- Families and social networks can celebrate gender diversity and challenge traditional gender norms.
- Embracing and valuing diverse gender identities helps create an environment where transgender individuals feel respected and affirmed.

7. Legal and Practical Support:

- Families and social networks can provide practical support in legal and administrative matters.
- Assisting with name and gender marker changes, navigating healthcare systems, and advocating for transgender-inclusive policies contribute to transgender individuals' well-being.

8. Continual Learning and Growth:

- Families and social networks should commit to ongoing learning and growth.
- Maintaining evolving terminology, understanding intersectionality, and challenging personal biases contribute to a supportive and inclusive environment.

By fostering acceptance, understanding, and support, families and social networks can play a transformative role in the lives of transgender individuals. Creating a safe and affirming environment that embraces gender diversity helps transgender individuals thrive, feel validated, and lead fulfilling lives.

Concise development of the topic "Transgender Rights and Legal Protections":

Chapter 16: Transgender Rights and Legal Protections

Transgender individuals face unique challenges related to discrimination, access to healthcare, and legal recognition. This chapter explores the importance of transgender rights and legal protections in promoting equality and ensuring the well-being of transgender individuals.

1. Anti-Discrimination Laws:

- Comprehensive anti-discrimination laws are essential to protect transgender individuals from discrimination in employment, housing, education, healthcare, and public accommodations.
- These laws aim to ensure equal treatment and opportunities for transgender individuals and prohibit discrimination based on gender identity or expression.

2. Legal Recognition of Gender Identity:

- Legal recognition of gender identity is crucial for transgender individuals to fully access their rights and benefits.
- Legal mechanisms such as gender marker change on identification documents, birth certificates, and passports enable transgender individuals to have documents that align with their gender identity.

3. Healthcare Access and Insurance Coverage:

- Transgender individuals often face barriers to accessing gender-affirming healthcare and insurance coverage for necessary medical interventions.

- Laws and policies that mandate inclusive healthcare coverage and remove exclusions for transgender-related care help ensure access to medically necessary treatments.

4. School and Workplace Protections:

- Transgender students and employees should be protected from discrimination and harassment in educational institutions and workplaces.

- Policies that explicitly prohibit discrimination based on gender identity allow students to use facilities that align with their gender identity and provide workplace accommodations to help create inclusive and safe environments.

5. Hate Crime Legislation:

- Hate crime legislation should include provisions that protect transgender individuals from violence, harassment, and targeted attacks.

- Enhancing penalties for crimes motivated by bias or prejudice based on gender identity helps deter violence and sends a strong message of societal condemnation.

6. Immigration and Asylum Protections:

- Transgender individuals fleeing persecution based on gender identity should be eligible for asylum and protected from discrimination in immigration processes.

- Policies that recognize the unique vulnerabilities faced by transgender immigrants and provide appropriate legal protections are essential.

7. Advocacy and Awareness:

- Advocacy efforts and raising awareness about transgender rights are crucial for advancing legal protections and societal acceptance.

- Transgender individuals, organizations, and allies are vital in advocating for legislative changes, promoting education, and challenging stereotypes and prejudices.

8. International Human Rights Standards:

- Transgender rights should be upheld following international human rights standards.

- International bodies and organizations play a critical role in advocating for the rights of transgender individuals and pressuring governments to enact and enforce protective legislation.

By enacting and enforcing laws that protect transgender individuals from discrimination, ensure legal recognition, and promote access to healthcare and education, society can foster inclusivity, equality, and respect for the rights and dignity of transgender individuals. Ongoing advocacy, education, and awareness are essential to drive positive change and advance transgender rights globally.

Chapter 17: Intersectionality: Exploring the Experiences of Transgender People of Color

Intersectionality recognizes that individuals have multiple social identities that intersect and influence their experiences. This chapter focuses on the unique challenges faced by transgender individuals of color and explores the concept of intersectionality in understanding their experiences.

1. Understanding Intersectionality:

- Intersectionality recognizes that gender identity and race intersect, shaping the experiences and challenges faced by transgender individuals of color.

- Transgender people of color may face compounded forms of discrimination, marginalization, and systemic barriers that arise from both their gender identity and their racial or ethnic background.

2. Multiple Forms of Discrimination:

- Transgender people of color often face discrimination from transphobia and racism.

- They may encounter disparities in healthcare access, employment opportunities, housing, education, and interactions with law enforcement due to overlapping prejudices.

3. Healthcare Disparities:

- Transgender people of color may encounter barriers to affirming and culturally competent healthcare.

- These barriers include limited resources, lack of provider awareness, language barriers, and systemic biases that impact their overall health and well-being.

4. Economic Inequality:

- Transgender people of color are more likely to experience economic challenges, including higher unemployment rates, underemployment, and poverty.
- Discrimination in the job market, limited educational opportunities, and systemic biases contribute to these disparities.

5. Violence and Harassment:

- Transgender people of color face increased risks of violence, harassment, and hate crimes.
- The intersection of transphobia and racism exposes them to higher levels of violence, including police brutality, intimate partner violence, and hate-motivated attacks.

6. Limited Representation and Advocacy:

- Transgender people of color often face limited representation in mainstream media, advocacy organizations, and policy-making spaces.
- Lack of representation hinders their ability to have their voices heard, influence policies that impact their lives, and access appropriate resources and support.

7. Community Resilience and Activism:

- Despite facing intersecting forms of discrimination, transgender people of color demonstrate resilience and engage in activism to create change.
- They form supportive communities, advocate for their rights, and work towards dismantling systems of oppression.

8. Intersectional Approaches and Allyship:

- Intersectional approaches are essential in addressing the experiences of transgender people of color.

- Allyship involves actively supporting and amplifying the voices of transgender people of color, advocating for policies that address intersecting forms of discrimination, and challenging racism and transphobia within society.

Understanding and addressing the unique challenges faced by transgender people of color requires an intersectional lens. It involves acknowledging and dismantling the intersecting systems of oppression that impact their lives, advocating for their rights, amplifying their voices, and promoting inclusive policies and practices that recognize their experiences and promote equity and justice.

Chapter 18: Media Representation and Its Impact on Transgender Individuals

Media representation plays a significant role in shaping societal perceptions and understanding of transgender individuals. This chapter explores the impact of media representation on transgender individuals and the importance of accurate and inclusive portrayals.

1. Stereotypes and Misrepresentation:

- Transgender individuals have often been subjected to harmful stereotypes and misrepresentations in the media.

- Portrayals that reinforce stereotypes, sensationalize transitions, or focus solely on the physical aspects can perpetuate stigma, misunderstanding, and discrimination.

2. Visibility and Representation:

- Positive and authentic representation in the media is crucial for the visibility and acceptance of transgender individuals.

- Media representation that showcases diverse transgender experiences, identities, and achievements can challenge stereotypes and promote understanding.

3. Humanizing Transgender Experiences:

- Accurate media representations humanize transgender experiences and highlight the commonalities shared with cisgender individuals.

- By depicting transgender characters with depth, complexity, and relatable storylines, the media can foster empathy and promote acceptance.

4. Influence on Public Perception:

- Media has a powerful influence on public perception and attitudes toward transgender individuals.
- Positive and inclusive media representations can reduce prejudice, discrimination, and violence against transgender individuals.

5. Amplifying Diverse Voices:

- Media platforms have a responsibility to amplify the voices of transgender individuals, particularly those from underrepresented communities.
- Centering diverse stories and experiences helps challenge monolithic narratives and fosters a more inclusive understanding of transgender identities.

6. Representation Behind the Scenes:

- Inclusive media representation involves on-screen portrayals and representation behind the scenes.
- Transgender individuals should be able to tell their stories, work in media production, and be involved in decision-making processes.

7. Media Education and Literacy:

- Promoting media education and literacy enables audiences to critically analyze and challenge harmful portrayals.
- Educating the public about transgender issues, terminology, and the impact of media representation can foster more informed and empathetic engagement.

8. Media Accountability and Ethical Reporting:

- Media organizations should prioritize ethical reporting practices and strive for accuracy, respect, and sensitivity in their coverage of transgender individuals.

- Promoting responsible journalism and holding media outlets accountable for misrepresentation or harmful depictions is crucial.

By promoting accurate, diverse, and inclusive media representations, the media industry can create a more accepting and understanding society for transgender individuals. Responsible media practices, authentic storytelling, and amplifying diverse voices are vital in challenging stereotypes, fostering empathy, and promoting positive social change.

Chapter 19: Religion and Transgender Issues: Perspectives and Conflicts

Religion significantly shapes beliefs, values, and societal attitudes toward gender identity and transgender individuals. This chapter explores the diverse perspectives and conflicts that arise at the intersection of religion and transgender issues.

1. Religious Perspectives:

- Different religious traditions hold varying views on gender identity and transgender experiences.
- Some religious denominations embrace transgender individuals as part of their faith community, affirming their identities and advocating for their rights.
- Others may have theological interpretations that present challenges or conflicts with transgender identities.

2. Scriptural Interpretations:

- Scriptural interpretations can be diverse within religious traditions, leading to varying understandings of gender and transgender issues.
- Different interpretations of religious texts can contribute to accepting or rejecting transgender individuals within religious communities.

3. Conflicting Beliefs and Values:

- Conflicts may arise when religious teachings or doctrines conflict with understanding gender identity and transgender experiences.

- Transgender individuals may face challenges finding acceptance and support within religious communities with more conservative views on gender.

4. Religious Discrimination and Stigmatization:

- Transgender individuals may experience discrimination and stigmatization within religious spaces due to gender identity.
- This can manifest in exclusion from religious rituals, denial of leadership positions, or social isolation within religious communities.

5. Intersectional Identities:

- Transgender individuals may also hold intersecting religious, ethnic, or cultural identities that influence their experiences.
- The interplay of these identities can present unique challenges and complexities in navigating transgender and religious communities.

6. Progressive Religious Movements:

- Some religious groups and denominations actively advocate for LGBTQ+ inclusion and affirm the rights and identities of transgender individuals.
- These progressive movements work towards reconciling religious beliefs with acceptance and support for transgender individuals.

7. Bridge Building and Dialogue:

- Dialogue and understanding between religious communities and transgender individuals are essential for fostering empathy and finding common ground.
- Interfaith dialogues, LGBTQ+-affirming religious organizations, and support from religious leaders can contribute to bridging the gap between religion and transgender issues.

8. Personal Faith Journeys:

- Transgender individuals may undergo personal faith journeys as they reconcile their gender identity with their religious beliefs.

- These journeys can involve finding affirming religious spaces, exploring spiritual practices outside traditional religious institutions, or reinterpreting religious teachings.

Navigating the complexities between religion and transgender issues requires open dialogue, respect for diverse beliefs, and a willingness to challenge and evolve understandings within religious communities. Balancing religious freedom and the rights and dignity of transgender individuals is an ongoing process that involves acknowledging and addressing the conflicts that arise and working towards greater inclusivity and acceptance.

Chapter 20: Debunking Myths: Addressing Misconceptions about Transgender People

Transgender individuals often face misconceptions and stereotypes contributing to their marginalization and discrimination. This chapter aims to debunk common myths and address misconceptions about transgender people, fostering a more accurate and compassionate understanding.

1. Myth: Being transgender is a choice.

- Reality: Gender identity is a deeply ingrained aspect of a person's identity and is not a choice.
- Scientific evidence supports the understanding that gender identity is a fundamental part of a person's being, separate from assigned sex at birth.

2. Myth: Transgender individuals are mentally ill or have a disorder.

- Reality: Being transgender is not a mental illness.
- While transgender individuals may experience mental health challenges related to societal stigma and discrimination, their gender identity is not a pathology.

3. Myth: Transgender people are confused or going through a phase.

- Reality: Gender identity is a valid and consistent aspect of a person's identity.
- Transgender individuals often undergo a process of self-discovery and self-acceptance, but their gender identity is not a phase or confusion.

4. Myth: Transitioning is purely cosmetic or for attention-seeking.

- Reality: Gender-affirming treatments and transitions are crucial for the well-being and mental health of many transgender individuals.
- Transitioning is a deeply personal and necessary process that involves aligning one's physical appearance with their internal sense of self.

5. Myth: Transgender people threaten public safety, especially in restrooms.

- Reality: No evidence supports the claim that transgender individuals threaten public safety.
- Transgender people have used public restrooms consistent with their gender identity for years without causing harm.

6. Myth: Transgender individuals are trying to deceive or trick others.

- Reality: Transgender individuals are not deceiving or tricking others by living authentically.
- Their gender identity is a sincere and honest expression of who they are, and they deserve respect and recognition.

7. Myth: Children are too young to understand their gender identity.

- Reality: Gender identity can manifest at a young age, and children can clearly understand their gender identity.
- Supporting transgender children in self-discovery and providing affirming environments is crucial for their well-being.

8. Myth: Transgender people are rare or abnormal.

- Reality: Transgender people exist in every culture and throughout history.
- While the exact prevalence is difficult to determine, transgender individuals are a part of the diverse human experience.

Challenging and debunking these myths is essential for creating a more inclusive and supportive society for transgender individuals. By promoting accurate information, fostering empathy, and challenging preconceived notions, we can break down barriers, reduce stigma, and ensure that transgender people are treated with dignity and respect.

TRANSGENDER JOURNEY

Chapter 21: Lack of Real Science: Examining Controversial Research and Debates

The field of transgender studies has faced debates and controversies regarding scientific research, which have sometimes contributed to misunderstandings and misconceptions. This chapter explores the challenges and controversies surrounding transgender research and highlights the need for rigorous and evidence-based science.

1. Understanding Scientific Inquiry:

- Science is a systematic process that aims to understand the world through observation, experimentation, and analysis.

- In transgender studies, rigorous scientific inquiry is crucial for advancing knowledge and challenging assumptions.

2. Methodological Challenges:

- Research in transgender studies faces unique methodological challenges, including sample sizes, participant access, and ethical considerations.

- These challenges can make conducting large-scale studies difficult or generalize findings to the broader transgender population.

3. Controversial Research:

- Some research studies in the past have been criticized for flawed methodologies, biased assumptions, or limited scope.

- These controversies have led to debates and conflicting findings, which can contribute to the lack of consensus in certain areas of transgender research.

4. The Importance of Peer Review:

- Peer review is a critical process in scientific research where experts evaluate the quality and validity of research studies.
- Peer-reviewed studies undergo rigorous scrutiny to ensure they meet scientific standards and contribute to the body of knowledge.

5. Evolving Understanding:

- Scientific understanding of transgender issues continues to evolve, reflecting advancements in research methodologies and increasing diversity of voices in the field.
- Ongoing research and robust scientific debates are necessary for refining our understanding of transgender experiences and identities.

6. Addressing Biases and Assumptions:

- Researchers need to be aware of their biases and assumptions that may influence the design and interpretation of their studies.
- Efforts should be made to incorporate diverse perspectives and voices, including those of transgender individuals, in research endeavors.

7. Building Consensus:

- Building consensus in transgender research requires open dialogue, collaboration, and replication of studies.
- Consensus is often reached through a cumulative process of multiple studies converging on similar findings and methodologies.

8. Centering Transgender Voices:

- Centering the experiences and voices of transgender individuals in research is crucial for obtaining accurate and meaningful insights.

- Collaborative and participatory research approaches can help ensure that research questions, methodologies, and interpretations align with the lived experiences of transgender people.

While controversies and debates exist within transgender research, it is important to recognize the value of rigorous scientific inquiry and the ongoing efforts to address limitations and biases. By promoting transparency, inclusivity, and robust research methodologies, we can foster a more accurate and nuanced understanding of transgender experiences.

Chapter 22: Transgender in the Workplace: Challenges and Progress

Transgender individuals face unique challenges in the workplace due to societal prejudices and misunderstandings. However, there has been progress in creating more inclusive work environments. This chapter explores the challenges faced by transgender individuals in the workplace and highlights the steps taken to promote inclusivity and equality.

1. Workplace Discrimination:

- Transgender individuals often experience discrimination and prejudice in hiring, promotion, and retention.
- Discrimination can manifest in various forms, including harassment, unequal treatment, and denial of workplace benefits.

2. Lack of Legal Protections:

- In many jurisdictions, legal protections for transgender individuals in the workplace are limited or absent.
- The absence of explicit protections can leave transgender employees vulnerable to discrimination and harassment.

3. Social Stigma and Bias:

- Prejudice and bias against transgender individuals contribute to a hostile work environment.
- Negative stereotypes and misconceptions can impact career advancement, workplace relationships, and job satisfaction.

4. Transitioning in the Workplace:

- Transitioning, and aligning one's gender presentation with gender identity, can pose challenges in the workplace.
- Transgender individuals may face anxiety and uncertainty about coming out and navigating changes in appearance or documentation.

5. Workplace Policies and Practices:

- Inclusive workplace policies that explicitly address gender identity and expression are crucial for supporting transgender employees.
- Policies related to dress

Chapter 23: Transgender and Sports: Fairness and Inclusion

Including transgender individuals in sports has sparked discussions and debates surrounding fairness, competition, and inclusivity. This chapter explores the complex issues surrounding transgender participation in sports and the efforts to promote fairness and inclusion.

1. Understanding Gender Identity:

- Gender identity is an individual's deeply held sense of gender, which may or may not align with the sex assigned at birth.

- Recognizing and respecting an individual's gender identity is essential in creating inclusive sporting environments.

2. Athletic Performance and Physiology:

- Concerns about the potential advantages or disadvantages of transgender athletes are often related to differences in physiology, strength, or performance.

- It is important to consider that athletic performance is influenced by factors beyond the sex assigned at birth, including training, genetics, and individual variation.

3. Fairness and Level Playing Field:

- Ensuring fairness in sports is a priority, as athletes deserve equitable competition opportunities.

- Policies and regulations should balance inclusivity with fair competition, considering factors such as hormone levels, length of hormone therapy, and other scientific guidelines.

4. Governing Body Policies:

- Many sports organizations and governing bodies have developed policies and guidelines regarding transgender participation.
- These policies aim to create a framework that addresses fairness concerns while promoting inclusion and respecting the rights of transgender athletes.

5. Science and Evidence-Based Approaches:

- Establishing fair policies and guidelines requires a scientific and evidence-based approach, considering the available research and expert input.
- Ongoing research and collaboration between sports organizations, medical professionals, and transgender athletes can contribute to more informed and fair policies.

6. Education and Awareness:

- Promoting education and awareness about transgender issues in sports is crucial for fostering understanding and empathy.
- Educating athletes, coaches, officials, and spectators can help dispel misconceptions and create a more inclusive sporting culture.

7. Transgender Athlete Experiences:

- Listening to and centering the experiences of transgender athletes is vital for informing policy development and understanding the challenges they face.
- Including transgender athletes in decision-making processes and creating support networks can contribute to more inclusive sports environments.

8. Evolving Policies and Practices:

- As scientific understanding and societal attitudes evolve, sports organizations must review and adapt their policies accordingly.
- Regular evaluation and policy updates can ensure that they reflect current knowledge and promote fairness and inclusion.

Finding a balance between fairness and inclusion in sports is an ongoing process that requires open dialogue, collaboration, and a commitment to understanding the unique experiences of transgender athletes. By considering the available scientific evidence, respecting gender identity, and creating inclusive policies, sports can become a more welcoming and equitable space for all athletes.

Chapter 24: Transgender Activism: Milestones and Current Movements

Transgender activism has played a crucial role in raising awareness, advocating for rights, and creating change for transgender individuals. This chapter explores the milestones and current movements within transgender activism, highlighting the progress made and ongoing challenges faced.

1. Stonewall Riots and Early Activism:

- The Stonewall Riots 1969, led by transgender women of color, marked a pivotal moment in LGBTQ+ activism, including transgender rights.
- Early transgender activists paved the way for future movements by challenging societal norms and advocating for visibility and acceptance.

2. Legal Milestones:

- Transgender activism has been instrumental in achieving legal milestones, such as the inclusion of gender identity in anti-discrimination laws and the recognition of transgender rights in various countries.
- Landmark court cases and legislative changes have expanded protections and rights for transgender individuals.

3. Visibility and Media Representation:

- Increased visibility and positive media representation have been central to transgender activism.

- Transgender activists and advocates have worked to challenge stereotypes, humanize transgender experiences, and promote understanding through storytelling and media engagement.

4. Transgender Day of Remembrance:

- Transgender Day of Remembrance, observed annually on November 20th, memorializes transgender individuals who have lost their lives due to violence and discrimination.
- This day serves as a reminder of the ongoing struggle for transgender rights and the need to address systemic violence and prejudice.

5. Intersectional Activism:

- Intersectionality recognizes that transgender activism intersects with other social justice movements, such as racial justice, feminism, and disability rights.
- Transgender activists have embraced intersectionality, advocating for the rights and well-being of transgender individuals within a broader context of social justice.

6. Healthcare Advocacy:

- Transgender activists have been at the forefront of advocating for improved healthcare access and quality for transgender individuals.
- Efforts have focused on addressing barriers to gender-affirming healthcare, combating insurance exclusions, and promoting transgender-inclusive medical guidelines.

7. Global Movements:

- Transgender activism extends beyond national borders, with global movements advocating for the rights and well-being of transgender individuals worldwide.
- International organizations, such as Transgender Europe (TGEU) and Global Action for Trans Equality (GATE), work towards promoting transgender rights on a global scale.

8. Ongoing Challenges and Future Directions:

- Despite significant progress, transgender activism faces challenges, including discrimination, violence, and a lack of legal protections in many regions.

- Future directions of transgender activism include addressing systemic inequalities, advocating for comprehensive transgender healthcare, and ensuring inclusive policies and practices in various sectors.

Transgender activism has made significant strides in advancing rights, visibility, and understanding. By amplifying transgender voices, challenging societal norms, and advocating for change, activists continue to shape a more inclusive and equitable world for transgender individuals.

TRANSGENDER JOURNEY

Chapter 25: Gender-Affirming Care for Non-Binary and Gender-Fluid Individuals

Gender-affirming care is not limited to binary transgender individuals; it also encompasses the unique needs of non-binary and gender-fluid individuals. This chapter explores the importance of gender-affirming care specifically tailored for non-binary and gender-fluid individuals, highlighting the challenges and progress in this area.

1. Understanding Non-Binary and Gender-Fluid Identities:

- Non-binary individuals identify outside the traditional gender binary of male and female, while gender-fluid individuals experience a fluidity in their gender identity over time.
- Recognizing and respecting these diverse gender identities is essential in providing appropriate and affirming care.

2. Individualized Approaches:

- Gender-affirming care for non-binary and gender-fluid individuals should be individualized, considering each person's unique gender identity and goals.
- Healthcare providers should engage in open, non-judgmental conversations to understand their patient's needs and preferences.

3. Inclusive Language and Documentation:

- Inclusive language and terminology are crucial in creating a safe and affirming healthcare environment.

- Healthcare providers should adapt their documentation and intake forms to include non-binary and gender-neutral options for gender identity and honor preferred names and pronouns.

4. Mental Health Support:

- Non-binary and gender-fluid individuals may face unique mental health challenges related to their gender identity, including gender dysphoria, identity exploration, and discrimination.
- Mental health professionals should provide affirming support, address gender-related concerns, and facilitate coping strategies to promote overall well-being.

5. Gender-Affirming Hormone Therapy:

- Hormone therapy can significantly influence gender affirmation for non-binary and gender-fluid individuals.
- Healthcare providers should work closely with patients to develop personalized hormone therapy plans that align with their goals and preferences.

6. Surgical Interventions:

- Some non-binary and gender-fluid individuals may desire surgical interventions to align their physical appearance with gender identity.
- Healthcare providers must discuss the range of surgical options available and ensure informed consent while considering each individual's specific goals and expectations.

7. Supportive Care Networks:

- Building supportive care networks is crucial for non-binary and gender-fluid individuals, who may face challenges navigating healthcare systems and finding inclusive providers.
- Collaborating with transgender and LGBTQ+ organizations can help create referral networks and promote access to gender-affirming care.

8. Ongoing Education and Training:

- Healthcare providers should engage in ongoing education and training to enhance their knowledge and understanding of non-binary and gender-fluid identities.

- By staying up-to-date with emerging research, best practices, and the evolving needs of non-binary and gender-fluid individuals, providers can offer more comprehensive and affirming care.

Addressing the unique needs of non-binary and gender-fluid individuals in gender-affirming care is essential for promoting their overall well-being and ensuring inclusive healthcare experiences. By adopting individualized approaches, using inclusive language, providing mental health support, and staying informed, healthcare providers can play a vital role in supporting the health and dignity of non-binary and gender-fluid individuals.

Chapter 26: Transgender Rights on a Global Scale

Transgender rights are a critical aspect of human rights and social justice. While progress has been made in many regions, the recognition and protection of transgender rights vary significantly globally. This chapter explores the status of transgender rights worldwide, highlighting the challenges faced and the ongoing efforts to promote equality and inclusion.

1. Regional Variations:

- Transgender rights and protections vary widely across different regions and countries.
- Some countries have comprehensive legal frameworks that protect transgender individuals from discrimination and provide access to gender-affirming healthcare, while others lack basic legal protections.

2. Legal Recognition:

- Legal recognition of gender identity is a fundamental aspect of transgender rights.
- Many countries have implemented legal procedures to enable transgender individuals to change their gender markers on identification documents, such as passports, identity cards, and birth certificates.

3. Anti-Discrimination Laws:

- Anti-discrimination laws protect transgender individuals from discrimination in various domains, including employment, housing, healthcare, and education.

- However, the scope and effectiveness of these laws vary across different countries.

4. Healthcare Access:

- Access to gender-affirming healthcare is a vital component of transgender rights.

- Inclusive healthcare systems should provide access to hormone therapy, gender-affirming surgeries, mental health support, and other necessary medical interventions.

5. Violence and Hate Crimes:

- Transgender individuals often face high violence, hate crimes, and targeted discrimination rates.

- Efforts to address and prevent violence against transgender individuals should be a central focus of global transgender rights advocacy.

6. Legal Recognition of Relationships:

- The legal recognition of relationships, including marriage and partnership rights, is crucial for transgender individuals and their families.

- Ensuring transgender individuals can form legally recognized relationships is important to achieving full equality.

7. Advocacy and Activism:

- Transgender rights movements and organizations are vital in advocating for legal reforms, raising awareness, and promoting societal acceptance.

- Transgender activists and allies work tirelessly to advance transgender rights on national and international platforms.

8. Global Initiatives:

- International organizations and initiatives, such as the United Nations Free & Equal campaign, focus on promoting LGBTQ+ rights, including transgender rights, globally.

- These initiatives raise awareness, share best practices, and advocate for policy changes to protect and promote transgender rights worldwide.

9. Intersectionality and Marginalized Communities:

- Transgender individuals from marginalized communities, such as people of color, indigenous populations, and refugees, face intersecting discrimination and are particularly vulnerable to human rights violations.

- Advocacy efforts must prioritize addressing the unique challenges faced by these individuals and ensure their inclusion in broader transgender rights movements.

While progress has been made in recognizing and protecting transgender rights globally, significant challenges persist. It requires ongoing advocacy, legal reforms, education, and societal transformation to achieve full equality for transgender individuals worldwide. By collaborating across borders, sharing best practices, and supporting grassroots activism, the global community can work together to advance transgender rights and create a more inclusive and equitable world for all.

Chapter 27: Mental Health Support for Transgender Individuals

Transgender individuals often face unique mental health challenges related to their gender identity and experiences of discrimination, stigma, and social exclusion. This chapter explores the importance of mental health support for transgender individuals and highlights the approaches and strategies to promote their well-being and resilience.

1. Understanding Mental Health Needs:

- Transgender individuals may experience gender dysphoria, anxiety, depression, and other mental health concerns related to their gender identity.
- Mental health professionals need to deeply understand transgender experiences and cultural competency to provide effective support.

2. Gender-Affirming Therapy:

- Gender-affirming therapy focuses on supporting transgender individuals in their gender identity exploration, acceptance, and alignment with their authentic selves.
- Therapists use affirmative and supportive approaches to help individuals navigate their gender journey and address mental health concerns.

3. Gender Dysphoria Treatment:

- Gender dysphoria, the distress experienced due to a mismatch between one's gender identity and assigned sex at birth, can significantly impact mental well-being.

- Mental health professionals can provide therapy and support with medical interventions, such as hormone therapy and gender-affirming surgeries, to alleviate gender dysphoria.

4. Culturally Competent Care:

- Mental health professionals should receive training in transgender cultural competency to provide sensitive and inclusive care.

- This includes understanding the unique challenges faced by transgender individuals, using appropriate language and terminology, and creating a safe and non-judgmental therapeutic environment.

5. Support Groups and Peer Networks:

- Support groups and peer networks are vital in providing validation, connection, and a sense of community for transgender individuals.

- These spaces allow individuals to share experiences, seek advice, and find support from others who understand their unique challenges.

6. Intersectionality and Multicultural Considerations:

- Recognizing the intersectional identities and experiences of transgender individuals is crucial in providing effective mental health support.

- Mental health professionals should consider the impact of race, ethnicity, culture, religion, and other intersecting factors on an individual's mental well-being.

7. Addressing Stigma and Discrimination:

- Stigma and discrimination can negatively affect the mental health of transgender individuals.

- Mental health professionals should help individuals develop coping strategies, resilience, and self-acceptance in the face of societal prejudice.

8. Collaboration with Medical Providers:

- Collaborating with medical providers in gender-affirming healthcare is essential for comprehensive mental health support.
- Coordination between mental health professionals and medical providers can ensure holistic care that addresses physical and mental well-being.

9. Ongoing Support and Follow-Up:

- Mental health support for transgender individuals should be an ongoing process, with regular check-ins, follow-up appointments, and access to crisis support when needed.
- Building long-term therapeutic relationships can help individuals navigate the challenges and celebrate the successes of their gender journeys.

Mental health support plays a critical role in the overall well-being of transgender individuals. By providing gender-affirming therapy, culturally competent care, support networks, and addressing stigma, mental health professionals can contribute to the resilience, self-acceptance, and empowerment of transgender individuals as they navigate their gender identities and experiences.

Chapter 28: The Role of Allies in the Transgender Rights Movement

Allies play a crucial role in supporting and advocating for the rights and well-being of transgender individuals. This chapter explores the significance of allies in the transgender rights movement, their responsibilities, and how they can create a more inclusive and equitable society.

1. Understanding Allyship:

- Allyship refers to individuals who support and stand up for marginalized communities, such as transgender individuals.

- Allies recognize and acknowledge the challenges faced by transgender individuals and actively work to promote their rights and well-being.

2. Educating Oneself:

- Allies should take the initiative to educate themselves about transgender identities, experiences, and issues.

- This includes understanding terminology, historical context, legal challenges, and the unique concerns and needs of transgender individuals.

3. Listening and Amplifying Transgender Voices:

- Allies should prioritize listening to transgender individuals, valuing their experiences, and amplifying their voices.

- Centering transgender voices in discussions about transgender rights ensures that their perspectives and needs are at the forefront of the movement.

4. Challenging Discrimination and Bias:

- Allies are responsible for challenging discrimination, bias, and harmful stereotypes about transgender individuals when they encounter them.
- This can be done through engaging in conversations, correcting misconceptions, and promoting understanding and acceptance.

5. Advocacy and Allyship:

- Allies can engage in advocacy efforts to promote transgender rights by participating in rallies, signing petitions, contacting elected officials, and supporting transgender-led organizations.
- Amplifying transgender stories and experiences through social media and other platforms can also contribute to broader awareness and acceptance.

6. Creating Inclusive Spaces:

- Allies can create inclusive spaces where transgender individuals feel safe, respected, and affirmed.
- This includes using inclusive language, respecting chosen names and pronouns, and advocating for inclusive policies in educational institutions, workplaces, and community settings.

7. Supporting Transgender Youth:

- Allies can be critical in supporting transgender youth by advocating for inclusive school policies, ensuring access to gender-affirming healthcare, and providing emotional support and validation.

8. Recognizing Intersectionality:

- Allies should recognize the intersecting identities and experiences of transgender individuals, particularly those from marginalized communities.
- This includes addressing racism, ableism, classism, and other forms of discrimination that transgender individuals may face.

9. Self-Reflection and Growth:

- Allies should engage in ongoing self-reflection and actively work to challenge their own biases and assumptions.
- Recognizing and learning from mistakes, being open to feedback from transgender individuals, and continually growing in allyship are essential.

Transgender rights movements greatly benefit from the support and involvement of allies. By educating themselves, listening to transgender voices, challenging discrimination, advocating for inclusive spaces, and recognizing intersectionality, allies can contribute to the ongoing struggle for transgender rights and create a more inclusive and equitable society.

Chapter 29: Future Directions: Advancements and Challenges

The transgender rights movement has significantly progressed in recent years, but many advancements and challenges remain. This chapter explores the future directions of the movement, highlighting areas for advancement and addressing the persistent challenges that transgender individuals continue to face.

1. Legal Protections:

- Advancement: Continued efforts are needed to secure comprehensive legal protections for transgender individuals, including anti-discrimination laws, legal recognition of gender identity, and access to gender-affirming healthcare.

- Challenge: Resistance to transgender-inclusive legislation and the need for broader societal acceptance pose challenges to achieving full legal equality.

2. Education and Awareness:

- Advancement: Increasing education and awareness about transgender identities and experiences can help dispel misconceptions, reduce stigma, and promote understanding and acceptance.

- Challenge: Resistance to inclusive education and dissemination of accurate information can hinder progress and perpetuate ignorance and discrimination.

3. Healthcare Access:

- Advancement: Improving access to gender-affirming healthcare, including hormone therapy, gender-affirming surgeries, and mental health support, is crucial for the well-being of transgender individuals.

- Challenge: Limited access to quality healthcare, affordability concerns, and lack of transgender-specific healthcare training for medical professionals pose challenges to equitable healthcare access.

4. Mental Health Support:

- Advancement: Strengthening mental health support for transgender individuals, including access to culturally competent therapists and support networks, can promote resilience and well-being.

- Challenge: Limited availability of transgender-affirming mental health resources and the need for the ongoing destigmatization of mental health issues within transgender communities are ongoing challenges.

5. Employment and Workplace Inclusion:

- Advancement: Creating inclusive workplaces that protect transgender individuals from discrimination, provide equal employment opportunities, and respect gender identity is crucial for economic empowerment.

- Challenge: Persistent workplace discrimination, wage gaps, and lack of inclusive policies hinder progress in achieving workplace equality for transgender individuals.

6. Transgender Youth Support:

- Advancement: Prioritizing the needs of transgender youth by providing inclusive schools, gender-affirming healthcare, mental health support, and protection from bullying and harassment is vital.

- Challenge: Resistance to transgender-inclusive policies in educational institutions, lack of comprehensive healthcare services for transgender youth, and increased vulnerability to mental health challenges remain significant.

7. Intersectionality and Marginalized Communities:

- Advancement: Recognizing and addressing the unique challenges faced by transgender individuals from marginalized communities, including people of color, immigrants, and disabled individuals, is crucial for achieving true equity.

- Challenge: The intersection of multiple forms of discrimination can lead to compounded challenges and requires comprehensive and inclusive solutions.

8. Global Advocacy:

- Advancement: Expanding global advocacy efforts to promote transgender rights, including sharing best practices, supporting grassroots movements, and addressing the specific needs of transgender individuals in different regions, can drive progress.

- Challenge: Varying legal and cultural contexts, resistance to change, and limited resources for global advocacy pose challenges to achieving widespread global recognition of transgender rights.

The future of the transgender rights movement lies in continued advancements and the collective efforts of individuals, communities, organizations, and policymakers. By addressing these challenges and working towards a more inclusive and equitable society, we can strive to ensure that transgender individuals are treated with dignity, respect, and equal rights in all aspects of life.

Conclusion: Towards a More Inclusive and Understanding Society

The journey towards a more inclusive and understanding society for transgender individuals requires ongoing commitment, education, and advocacy. Throughout this book, we have explored various aspects of transgender issues, including definitions and concepts, historical perspectives, human freedom, gender identity development, mental health challenges, medical interventions, legal protections, and the vital role of allies and activism. By addressing these topics, we hope to contribute to a deeper understanding of transgender experiences and foster empathy and acceptance.

Transgender individuals deserve to live authentically, free from discrimination, stigma, and marginalization. They can access healthcare, education, employment opportunities, and legal protections without fear of prejudice. Achieving this vision requires collective action from individuals, communities, organizations, and policymakers.

It is crucial to recognize that transgender rights are human rights. Every person should have the freedom to express their gender identity and to be treated with dignity and respect. This includes acknowledging the importance of self-identification, affirming pronouns, and chosen names, and providing gender-affirming healthcare options.

Creating a more inclusive society also involves addressing intersecting forms of discrimination based on race, ethnicity, socioeconomic status, and disability. Transgender individuals from marginalized communities often face compounded challenges and require targeted support and advocacy.

Education and awareness play vital roles in dismantling misconceptions and promoting understanding. By disseminating accurate information about transgender identities and experiences, we can challenge stereotypes, reduce stigma, and foster empathy. This education should start early, including in schools, to promote a more inclusive and accepting generation.

The journey towards a more inclusive society is not without its challenges. Resistance, prejudice, and systemic barriers can hinder progress. However, we can create real change through continued advocacy, policy reform, and grassroots movements.

As we conclude this book, let us remember that the fight for transgender rights is ongoing. It requires an ongoing commitment to challenge and dismantle systems of oppression, create inclusive spaces, and advocate for equal rights and opportunities. Together, we can work towards a society that embraces and celebrates the diversity of gender identities, ensuring that transgender individuals can live their lives authentically, with dignity, and in full equality.

In our collective efforts, we can build a future where transgender individuals are fully recognized, supported, and celebrated as valuable global community members. Let us strive towards a society that embraces differences, promotes understanding, and upholds the fundamental principles of human rights and equality for all.

www.ingramcontent.com/pod-product-compliance
Lightning Source LLC
Chambersburg PA
CBHW072031230526
45466CB00020B/1521